Rehab the Mind, Revive the Body
Foundations for Healing

© DR. JUSTIN C. LIN

Copyright © 2014 by Rehab and Revive Physical Therapy Inc.
All rights reserved. This book or any portion thereof may not be
reproduced, stored in a retrieval system, or transmitted in any form by
any means, electronic, mechanical, photo-copying, recording, or
otherwise, without the express written permission of the {book owners}
except for the use of brief quotations in a book review.

Printed in the United States of America
First Printing, 2014
ISBN 978-0-9907134-1-8

Rehab and Revive Books, a subsidiary of Rehab and Revive Physical
Therapy Inc.
3002 Dow Avenue, Suite 502
Tustin, CA 92780
www.rehabandrevive.com
Copyright © 2014 Dr. Justin C. Lin
All rights reserved.

ISBN: 0990713415

TABLE OF CONTENTS

Dedication	v
Foreword – Shifting the Paradigm	vii
Introduction – Old Habits Die Hard	xi
Chapter One – Dislocation: The Origin of Possibilities	1
A Lesson in Empowerment	13
Chapter Two – Bundle of Nerves: Unraveling the Hidden Pain	17
Rehab and Revive: A Practice is Born	31
Chapter Three – Headstrong: Trust the Process	35
Chapter Four – Shortcuts: The Case for Prevention	49
Chapter Five – Choose Life: Leaving the Cycle of Pain	61
Candid – An Interview With Gregg Johnson, Co-Founder of the Institute of Physical Art	73

KJELD,
   THANK YOU FOR
YOUR TRUST & LOVE
TO THE PROCESS.
   WELCOME TO THE
CLUB.
   LIVE EMPOWERED,
   CHOOSE THE REINA!

DEDICATION

It is my honor to dedicate this effort to all of my patients for allowing me to be a witness to some of the most triumphant moments of your lives. Your choices to live inspire me every day. I am eternally indebted to my many mentors and teachers whose guidance in this pursuit has helped make my dream a reality. And I am humbled by my parents, Luisa and Oliver, keeping their most important promise, and by the support of my sister, Frances, who has been my confidante throughout life's adventure.

FOREWORD
Shifting the Paradigm

"We cannot change our past. We cannot change the fact that people act in a certain way. We cannot change the inevitable. The only thing we can do is play on the one string we have, and that is our attitude." – Charles Swindoll

Counterintuitive mindsets tend not to absorb quickly into our psyches; rather, we fight against their effects, cynics who waste hours, years, or even lifetimes. Rehab and Revive seems straightforward enough; physical therapy is just that—rehabilitation and, we hope, a revival. However, my intuition (or perhaps my experience) focused on a single, twofold goal: rehabilitate the mind and revive the body.

Doesn't it make more sense to rehab the body and *then* revive the mind? This is the typical mindset of our culture—treating the symptom and not the root problem. My philosophy diverges here, mainly because I spent most of my life trying to dump my efforts into the perfect physique and the ideal diet. I have only come to find after these often frivolous and wasted commitments that these efforts are just that: skin-deep. I learned that my efforts to invest in a body that is constantly requiring an aesthetic upkeep was an endless pit, and I wasn't entirely happy with the superficial results. Like most athletic people, six-packs, 20-mile runs, and muscle pain consumed me like a fanatic. It took the pain to provoke change, and higher numbers of reps didn't do the trick.

I have always contended that mindless movements are useless movements, and the same could be said about a mindless life. Awareness is key. In order to create *meaningful* change, we need to risk being vulnerable and unattached from our preconceived fears and notions. In order to create *lasting* change, we need to work hard to achieve the *right* goal.

The road to good health is truly a process that is part of an endless cycle. When you complete one cycle, another unknown barrier and self-limiting belief will be staring you in the face, needing to be overcome. There is no way to deceive yourself. Physical artists (healers) can only be your leg for so long—one day you'll have to claim it as your own because, if truly good health is part of your plan, you alone are going to have to clear the hurdles of life. Reaching the bottom of the barrel is often a lonely, frustrating experience. Despite that darkness, however, climbing into the light and rising to the challenge seems so much harder.

When achieving all the limitless possibilities in life, we must tap into the endless and inspirational potential of our minds. One thing you may find there is that, if you are ravenous for a better life, rising like a phoenix becomes infinitely easier. In fact, you will find that thriving—and not merely surviving—is our natural state of being.

When I started my healing journey, it was arduous; I had to accept my reality instead of desperately holding onto a fantasy, which then allowed the vision to move forward in life, happiness, and health. Valuing this mental shift in thought was what truly began the process of evolution for my body. Rehabilitating my thoughts was step one. My body simply reaped the benefits of revitalization from a mind well trained.

Times and characters have been changed to protect the identities of those whose stories are shared in this book, but the stories are real. Healing, transformation, and hope are the most universal of human experiences. Please invite them into your hearts, as they are cherished in mine. I hope you come to find that incentives for growth begin and end with the mind, because a strong will must tend toward the correct path. Facing challenges with courage and character requires you to don your cape, and I am here to shine a light on the strength of your internal power. I am convinced that you will all learn to rehab your mind and revive your body.

With all my gratitude,

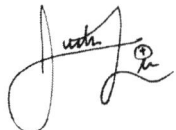

INTRODUCTION
Old Habits Die Hard

I am a Frankenstein, the stitched-together creation of too many doctors with too many scalpels, a discombobulated embodiment of the American medical system. Twenty injuries, seven surgeries, and one leg that could barely bear my weight—I was a prisoner of my body, with a shackled mind to boot. When did my body remove itself so entirely from my mind? This epidemic is wholly incongruent with the grain of nature, yet such a habit of natural beings: disassociation between what drives us and what moves us, when, in fact, they should be one and the same. The confluence between my brain and body was simply missing—a pattern typical of most. Born healthy, move incorrectly, suffer immensely, go under the knife, limp slowly, medicate aggressively, rinse and repeat—the medical system has created a seamless (if they go through the belly button!) model of physical training and subsequent healing.

We are taught, from birth, incorrect walking patterns, which lead to erroneous physical training in sports that result in severe deformations in our physical structure, many of which thoroughly impede our movements and, ultimately, our lives. Yet how is this possible? We are a nation of healers, not a nation of preventers, doctors of medicine whose very professions are founded upon an oath of ethics and honesty. In fact, I can't seem to find a single line in the hundreds of medical textbooks that I studied dedicated to pills or exploratory surgery, terms that are now common nomenclature for patients. How far we are from the healthcare system that aided our healing instead of glamorizing our maladies to augment the nobility of the profession?

I was under the impression when I first ventured into the medical profession that doctors were simply moneymakers with a pharmacy. I saw that they complicated our maladies to such an extent that we had no choice but to believe them: ADHD, chronic blood pressure, internal something or other, and the list goes on. If patients were made to feel that the only conduit to healing was vis-à-vis their doctor (meaning pills and surgery), then the medical profession accomplished two things: bamboozling patients into fear and making money by "treating" their fear. There are many conditions that require extensive medical intervention, and doctors do a phenomenal job making progress in helping our society, but more and more, these treatments lack one vital component: the participation of the patient. How can I expect my patients to heal if they aren't taught how? This is a travesty for the powerless persons who rely on medicine, but it also gave me pause as to who else was powerless in the system, and it dawned on me: doctors themselves are inert spectators, despite their acute and extensive education. They have not been trained in the art of healing, but rather in the clinic of pharmaceutical companies. By diagnosing the symptoms and not reaching toward the origin, solutions become band-aids. The true essence of medicine is to serve the patient first, not to satiate the ego of a corporate medical entity.

Unsurprisingly, we have learned to live within these confines, brainwashed in both our physical movements and our perception of reliance. The medical system has impressed upon the American public the single most detrimental untruth: that we are incapable of healing ourselves. This pervasive mentality starts in the brain, as most dependent behaviors do—the Rule of 21 substantiates this claim. See, repeating an action or a series of sentiments 21 times forms a habit, a tendency that in turn trains our minds to perform a series of actions that our bodies follow. Unfortunately, these habits often result in faulty physical movements. Yet, just like water, the body wants to flow easily and naturally, unencumbered by habits and fears, in total control of our surroundings, living without a need to react to external factors. The origin of these learned behaviors is wholly incongruent with our natural state of competency and often overrides our ability to properly adapt our mind to our body.

Perhaps I couldn't divorce my pains from my choice to pursue physical therapy as a profession, or maybe I couldn't justify practicing this powerless medicine to myself, prescribing pills to numb the pain, removing body parts to cover my bases, or simply bypassing the source and treating the symptoms. Perhaps my personal trauma propelled my innate need to delve into the depths of pain, analyzing the source, prodding, poking, and pushing toward the root. I could not in good faith reconcile using band-aids...maybe it was the ego of my inner Sherlock Holmes, or maybe I just felt the silently deafening cries for help from those who came to me as a last resort. And in the same vein that I treat my patients, I strive to understand my motives. This is the purest form of medical practice—staying ceaselessly curious, being relentlessly hungry for new knowledge, seeking innovative insights to one end only: healing the sick, preventing pain, and empowering others.

As each new patient enters my practice, they simultaneously access my mind, sometimes as unresolved problems that need solutions, sometimes as barriers that must be shattered. And the relationship becomes symbiotic; as they come to me as the last resort following a string of failed attempts with other doctors, I, too, am healed by their tenacity to overcome their struggles. But what makes me their last resort? Desperation has that effect—we exhaust our preconceived notions, hedging our bets on doctors who read from scripts: "Surgery, steroids, pills." Many fall into the trap, myself included, simply because the despondency is too much to bear. And old habits die hard—just ask your knees. Those who choose not to partake in the profitable and defenseless American medical system search for alternatives, and the few options that arise don't meet our standards for "real" medical care. The Goldilocks dilemma arises: this doctor is too surgery-happy (Western medicine perception), that doctor lights incense in the treatment room (Eastern medicine perception), but which one will heal me?

This is where Rehab and Revive comes in, a harmonious blend of Western science and Eastern touch, bridging the gap between all that hurts and all that helps. Retrain the brain, recalibrate the body, revive life. That's a pill that I can swallow.

1

DISLOCATION
The Origin of Possibilities

He picks him up gingerly, transferring Lucas from his wheelchair to the treatment table, and it is more akin as a journey from being in jail to having wings. "Positioning is key," the Doctor mutters under his breath, adjusting the geometries from hip to elbow, from his hand to Lucas's foot, seeking a perfect symmetry of proportions and alignments, even in preparation. Lucas makes an emphatic thumbs-up gesture, and the clarity of sentiment juxtaposes entirely with the contractions of his body, twitching, gesticulating, spastically uncontrolled. Cerebral palsy overwhelms his body and mind, full of short movements and disjointed almost-connections, yet Lucas is anything but disabled. He is keen, hilarious, a flirt, focused, determined: he is the definition of grit. No movement exists that he does not try, fails to match, or refuses to participate in, despite his palpable pain.

And it reveals itself. "We need to put the body in neutral," the Doctor states. "His hypersensitivity to the environment requires that I rely on micro-cues in every movement." And Therapy Room 2 is filled with sensitive glances, from his assistant, whose trained yet reticent hands supplement when needed, to Lucas's mother, "Coach", whose intimate knowledge of every gesticulation is evident in the creased corners of her bright eyes. Coach, mother, lioness, undefeated by the spasm of her other heart. A trainer even in simple glances, she doesn't observe—she visually controls in cues and coos to her son, the fighter.

Our current perception of Lucas's motor limitations is oft confused as a motor deficiency when, in fact, his extreme motor sensitivity dominates his neural pathways—to light, to mood, to sound, to aura, to thought, an uncontrolled and evident reaction to the atmosphere. Perhaps his absolute awareness of the unseen environment overwhelms his computing capacity, and in those moments, Lucas can't connect.

"Eyes over here!" she snapped, and Lucas returned from whatever reverie brought a grin to his face. He cried in pain as his hip was adjusted, his malady addressed. Five years before, powerless doctors performed uneducated acts, without witnesses, and dislocated his hip with a violence that stole his mobility, his freedom, his bikes up steep trails. This violation of movement sparked a distrust that didn't suit Lucas; a countenance of exuberance has no place alongside the anguish of ache. Because of his injury, his quality of life suffered, and gains that had taken a lifetime of determination deteriorated rapidly, day after day, contraction by contraction, and he became shorter. His body found a position that produced the least amount of pain, yet contorted his once-nimble frame into a series of twists and turns from head to toe.

The sudden and speedy thoughts course themselves across the randomness in my mind like a frightened school of fish. "What can I do? What will I do? I've never treated a patient with cerebral palsy. Take a breath...breathe...just think. What makes sense? Does it even make sense?" My pulse matches Lucas's intensity, and we beat together, rhythmic, chaotic, frantic.

This compensatory behavior is typical of the body, but only if it is stressed, is weak, or lacks control over or the right modulating of senses. I must choose a path that takes compensation out of the game, but how I can persuade the body to detour from that ease?

Water chooses the path of least resistance—or does it create the path of least resistance? I suppose it doesn't matter, as long as the sentiment shines through: ease is key. The body, like water, avoids obstacles as often as possible: the natural state of our physical being tries diligently to circumvent pain, from our first movement through the birth canal to our posture at our desks. Our pain receptors send clear messages to our brain— "Avoid! Deflect! Stop! Go!"—in an effort to make efficient use of our movements. So when pain does occur, either from acute injury or chronic habits, we are caught off guard; the body simply recoils and retreats, rendering our injured parts useless until healed. When I ripped my rotator cuff in high school, the pain forced my movements to cease, yet, like most people, I didn't listen to my body. In an effort to rule the world at the ignorant age of 17, and with a promising baseball career looming in my future, I forced mind over matter, and I kept pursuing my training, faster, harder, and stronger. Yet, when broken or misaligned, I was forced eventually to come to a complete stop or be sucked under the growing wave, and my body suddenly had a mind of its own.

Unable to ignore our injuries, we start the unconscious process of compensation, forming an awkward balance between how our body should move and how it can move. The goal? Pain avoidance. As I learned the hard way (as many do), avoiding obstacles only renders us less capable of conquering them when they inevitably rise again. Contorting into unhealthy positions and patterns is our natural tendency in this cycle of inflicting injury and then subsequently counterbalancing to sidestep the discomfort.

In my case, loading the pain onto various parts of my body that were not equipped to handle the extra stress only exacerbated my localized injury. Overuse, incorrect form, and even—as in Lucas's case—natural deformity in physical ability can all contribute to the downward cycle of injury, which in and of itself is simply a symptom of a much deeper root of maladies in the body.

Interestingly, I believe that we tend to develop these strategies of compensation based upon one simple and extraordinary fact: we've run out of options. Our body is simply down to no other choice than the one that augments the harm, and obviously, that is a terrible position to come to. The pain doesn't disappear; it only migrates from limb to limb, rendering each one weaker and more incapable, and it eventually circles right back to the origin.

This eventuality approaches the point of no return for many people, as it did for me. Our body contracts, our nerves compress, and our "creative compensatory" patterns solidify. Self-limitations dictate our capabilities, shrinking our world of freedom and choice.

Incongruent with our philosophy on choice is our innate fear of pain; our bodies ironically cling to negative compensation *routes. Lucas taught me a vital lesson in this mentality: when we are faced with fear, our inclination is to crouch, making our bodies smaller, contracting our muscles, and disengaging our minds from our bodies. The result? An absolute unawareness of our smallness, a disassociation from neuron to joint, a cacophony of spastic movements that in reality makes us less capable of healing in any real way.*

So Lucas twists on the table, a compressed series of joints that have swung too far off the pendulum of over-activity to underutilization, a lack of balance that exists as a caricature of his capabilities. Beads of sweat form and collect on my forehead, a sign that even the smallest doubt could impair my patient further. But seeds of doubt threaten me every day; how can I truly aid the injured when my body is still recovering? Oh yes—the process, the building blocks of clarity, composition, and calm, from limb to mind. I inhale slowly, deeply, methodically. My own body organizes itself, brain to body, blocks of stabilized power that ready themselves to finally move Lucas from point A to point B. I have but one choice: let's get back to square one. Let's get back to neutral.

"Touch your tongue to your teeth. Come on, Lucas, press the tip of your tongue to the roof of your mouth." The Doctor leans over a twisted Lucas, his body aligned against the patient's frame, one leg braced against the wall. He wheedles again: "Try and touch your tongue all the way to the back of your teeth, just like you're drinking through a straw." Lucas grins through the commands. His body reacts, first not at all, then spastically, then—finally—seamlessly. Typically snapped back to his spine, his neck now begins to lengthen, shifting his shoulders forward, straightening the arch of his back, pushing his hip down, a harmonious dance that calls the body to action. The coil begins to unwind itself, and the coach chimes in.

"Lucas, baby, just like you're trying to suck on a straw, keep it up!" And he does. In perfect symmetry, his hip aligns, and the Doctor, panting above him, pushes harder. The assistant with ready arms watches in anticipation, her years of schooling fighting against what her eyes witness: movement that has generated from the mind.

The years of struggle against the self have dictated Lucas's movements, and his body cannot hide the patterns that are written in every jerk. "How is this helping?" the incredulous assistant asks. "How is he suddenly so relaxed?" The question hangs in the air, and no solution seems logical. Another question, this time from the Doctor, a frustratingly innocuous query: "Did Lucas breastfeed?" The coach, with a quizzical expression, responds in the negative, and the Doctor nods, satisfied—yet his bated breath does not subside. At his behest, the observers place their tongues to their teeth, "like sucking through a straw." And the answer reveals itself profoundly and suddenly, with ramifications that reverberate from the womb to walking.

Touching your tongue to the roof of your mouth imitates the most human of motions—breastfeeding, a movement that follows us from the moment of birth. The muscles of the neck strengthen in this form, a neuromuscular education that generates life-long patterns of mobility. Those muscles and their subsequent strengthening patterns aid in our daily lives. To achieve this movement correctly, the body must come to a neutral position, lengthening fully from tongue to toe. The most primal of human acts prepares us for the most basic of human needs—movement. We can never ignore the origin; we can never bypass the root for the symptom because ease comes so easily.

His back is straighter, grimaces transform into grins, and Lucas raises his arms in victory. The feeling is contagious. Smiles spread like wildfire around Therapy Room 2, and the Doctor pushes harder. "Push me back," he instructs, placing pressure on Lucas's knee. "We need to reeducate your brain to accept these movements as natural."

"Come on, Lucas, push him back!" intone the onlookers in quiet unison. "Push him back!" screams Lucas's furious mind.

"Push me back!" commands the Doctor again. "Come on, Lucas, push me back!" Their energy is palpable in the room, from student to teacher, power to power, arm to arm. But Lucas cannot push back. The movements don't translate; his body needs help. He can't do it alone.

I can't pinpoint when I become the patient. Sometimes I shift for just a moment, extending a movement for my patient that seems just beyond their reach. With Lucas it seems that I shift seamlessly from my body to his, an interaction that occurs without conscious thought, initiated only by an unspoken bond. I will him to move, to push, to become long, and I feel his eyes responding, his brain initiating, his will focusing. Yet his body fails to listen, overwhelmed by the signals, too sensitive to the pressure, aware of my frustration. I need him to move and respond. I don't intend to fail him. The reeducation of his neural connections courses through my synapses, as my knee jerks when his fails, and so I push for him. Perhaps our energies unite, or perhaps the atmosphere becomes one of a calm victory, or perhaps Lucas is done testing me, but we begin to move together. First minutely, then in moments, and finally in motions.

My injury calls to me in these moments of absolute powerlessness, when neither my surgeon nor my body responded to my will. Days spent lamenting my unfortunate inability to connect my torn rotator cuff, stitched together with a nut here and a bolt there, here a screw, there a pin, everywhere a band-aid. It was all my doctor could do for me, and all I could do for myself. The utter inability to control my movements tormented me to no end. I was a prisoner shackled to my inability, and no amount of reason, scalpels, or Morphine injected activity back into my veins. Who had the power to heal me? When would 10% of my original capacity in movement return to 50% or 70%, or—dare I say it—100%?

That's where desperation met resolve, and I made my first visit to physical therapy. It was exhausting, basic, and painful. It called into action both muscle and mind together, and for the first time after two years of absolute pain, a familiar sensation tingled in me: hope. For six months, I clung to the feeling, rigorously demanding that my body marry my brain, slowly and methodically empowering the once-severed connections to reform, reset, renew. If this was rehabilitation, it worked for me. And at 90% restored capacity, I did what any 19-year-old would do—I stepped back up to the plate.

I noticed that the therapy required something from me that I saw in the therapists' movements—active participation. I learned that, if I couldn't move alone, I had a partner who would move for me, encouraging my limbs to relearn their lost capacities, engaging my motor controls, and empowering me to manage what was once mine—myself. In meeting and matching my patients at the precise level where they can bend, break, and shatter even their own preconceived limiting beliefs, and then guide them to this decision, I must understand the background story of each journeyman that walks through my door. Earning their trust is key to their growth.

It is perhaps the violence of the first movement that is the most difficult to control, a convulsive pop of energy that releases more than the joint; it frees the mind from the prison of pain. Because it truly is a prison in which our lives are brought to a standstill, and our baselines of our own selves diminish. In my case, this meant that I couldn't pursue a life that I had prepared for—a career in baseball and a future in sports. My injuries squashed those dreams and altered my reality, forcing a change in perspective that I ferociously fought against, until I ultimately overcame. In Lucas's case, his hip injury distorted his hard-earned physical baselines—and physical freedom is vital for a young man with cerebral palsy. He was a prisoner in a wheelchair, which became his legs, his hips, his body. It was time for the body to regain its legs, and so I made the choice to extend his movement into my own, becoming his body until he was strong enough to stand on his own.

The moment of truth arrived, and I urged him on: "Push me back, buddy. Come on, push me back." And as I felt his muscles tense, his joints stabilize, and his eyes squint in dedication to his goal, and as his small frame gave me an inch, I took it a mile: Five years to the day since his injury, Lucas rode his bike one mile up the hill at his parents' home—and he did it all by himself.

A Lesson in Empowerment
Give a man a fish, and you'll feed him for a day. But teach and a man to fish, and you'll feed him for a lifetime.

My first lesson in self-empowerment came to me in my early teenage years, when acne had taken residence on my face. Like every other teenager, I was mortified—this was unacceptable and intolerable, and pills were the cure. Accutane® was the drug of choice, a favorite to burn away the existence of scars that didn't belong, but the dollar cost wasn't the only high price. This caustic healing agent burnt my peers' faces, but we were forced to choose between the lesser of two evils, because we wanted a pimple-free face, and *NOW*.

It was highly misleading, because the product caused one simple result: an utterly dry and burnt complexion that couldn't harbor acne-causing bacteria, let alone sustain a modicum of vital moisture. In essence, it simply destroyed the balance. But I was a kid, and I couldn't care less about how I achieved clear skin so long as I did. The time had come for my branding into adulthood, and so I ventured to the nearest dermatologist, ready to be cured. Just my luck—I was assigned Dr. Mark.

I walked in, expecting to walk out with a prescription for Accutane®. I came out with no prescription, but with a large dose of something that I didn't want or expect: empowerment. I had one task—don't touch my face. It was a letdown of epic proportions.

I was at first flabbergasted by his recommendation. "I'll get your face looking better, but do me a favor, Justin—don't touch it for six weeks," he said, and then left the room. With outstretched arms as though I was expecting a bounty of gifts from Santa, I was looking for him to write a prescription and drop it into my waiting hands.

He exited the exam room, content with his advice. After about five confused minutes, I packed up my belongings and walked out to the reception desk. The receptionist confirmed my fear: "No, he didn't leave you a prescription...," but informed me that he wanted to see me back in six weeks. Three hundred dollars and a wasted hour later, my pimple-laden face and I trudged back home, angry, a petulant child with no understanding.

But that's the thing: our society expects to be given some kind solution by our providers, one that most typically arrives in the form of a pill, shot, or surgery. Leaving with nothing... what did it mean? I obviously had no power over my acne!

I did leave with something else, though, however undiscovered and intangible at that moment—I got my first lesson in being an active participant in my healing. The "medicine" I was prescribed was simple: don't touch my face for six weeks.

Over the next week, angry and bitter about the appointment, I would come to find that I touched my face a lot. I found that I touched my visage in class, in front of friends, in the library, after touching food, after shaking hands, etc. I did it so much that I counted that I did it once every two to three minutes of my waking day. I was suddenly aware of my actions, my habits, and the results.

I decided to stop making myself a victim and, instead of picking my face, I picked the option to start controlling my movements. Stopping myself from touching my face over the next few weeks was one of the most difficult "addictions" I have ever overcome. Changing habits, no matter what how nominal they seem to be, is an uphill battle, both internally and externally.

In order to satisfy the requirements of successfully breaking a habit, you need to fight instantly gratifying behavior, fear, judgment, ego, and attachments. Many would rather call it a day and stick their tails between their legs than endure the journey to the other side, stewing in negative patterns rather than conceding to change.

Once I broke loose from those shackles and escaped the sirens telling me to continue touching my face, magic happened. Six weeks later, my face was only 25% afflicted. I decided to pay Dr. Mark a visit, just to tell him that it took some serious courage for him to illuminate my real "disease"—my addiction to mindless habits. His challenge was met, and what ensued was a small dose of mild antibiotics, which sealed the deal in about another month. After only three visits, I was cured! I got a lesson in myself, a habit I no longer have, and a clean face to boot.

Dr. Mark told me that it was my chance to illustrate that I was strong enough to resist such tempting habits. He admitted that he would have eventually let me have my way with Accutane® if I couldn't resist myself. After the experience with overcoming my engraved tendencies, I feel so sad for those who are only offered that route, when such a simple (albeit tough) solution could be prescribed. By forgoing the "modern" method of constant monitoring of my face of this drug, at $300 a visit, Dr. Mark declined to fatten his wallet, knowing that he could have given me—the patient—a chance to prove that I didn't need medicine.

What good is giving someone blood pressure and pain drugs so quickly, like they're off-the-shelf candy? What good is all of this if they weren't offered or urged enough by their practitioners to make self-changes? What good is all of this if no one knew they had the *ability* to make self-changes in a limited-belief world?

What I received from Dr. Mark was pure medicine, and I reveled in it as the beneficiary of this style of practice—the kind of medicine that put me first, giving me not only what I needed, but also what I wanted. This lesson now governs how I manage my own patients.

2

BUNDLE OF NERVES
Unraveling the Hidden Pain

It crept, much like the clutter that starts in the corner of your desk, compiling odds and ends of forgotten papers, injuries, and bills. In sight but out of mind—at first it doesn't seem like much, and your eyes pass over it, noticing, but not discerning, until one day when you look and actually see, and you're horrified at the mess that has taken over your room.

For Eve, the pain had existed in perpetuity. Ankle soreness was familiar, a relic of an injury she didn't tend to. So were headaches, "in-laws" who stopped by without notice, and, as time passed, even those weren't a surprise, and she learned to bear with them. It was a low bar that didn't leave much room for less, but one can always fall.

Eve expected new pains beyond bruises and the odd strain or jammed knuckle, and, despite her high-impact choice of activity—martial arts—the apparent inevitability of her impending injury loomed. She learned to cope, adding it to the chorus of wounds that continued to exist. Bruises from the expected bully, hitting with a familiar cacophony of pain - vibrating, pulsating, numbing. It was hopeless to hope. But added to both were aches that were unexpected and inexplicable: these were the most unnerving. And even here she learned to duck the distress, bobbing and weaving to evade the inevitable, yet random fists caught her, and her wind was knocked out.

She ignored sensations of numbness and tingling that were vague at first, as well as a sudden sharp throb that accompanied the shoulder ache, a throb that literally stole her breath as the reverberations moved throughout her spine. Her body resolved itself against these, dulling, numbing, and intermittent. A year later, the headache started thumping like a loud bass drum and simply never stopped. With no explanation for it, she became accustomed to the constant, buzzing pressure in her skull. Zoom forward another two years, and a glance in the mirror revealed a slightly deformed rib cage, again, seemingly out of the blue. Hers was a face that she could no longer recognize—evidence of her being ebbing away. But her body had no recourse this time. The bully had left a scar.

❖

"Stuck, just stuck!" I muttered to myself. "She seems so reserved, out of options, just stuck!" I kept these observations to myself, because sharing them didn't seem prudent. She was hidden in herself, unwilling to speak, not wanting to be touched, scared to share. I had to adapt to coax answers from her by illuminating myself. True, I can be hardheaded at times, too proud and too direct—tough love to my patients to hurry along their journey. But this patient wasn't going to accept that type of healing. I couldn't ask for her involvement; I had to create an environment that encouraged it to divulge itself in bits and pieces. The journey was hers, and taking myself out of the equation was the only way to gain her trust.

I can't place the moment, but the memory is alive and well—10 years old, a boy with the elastic waistband shorts (my mom affectionately coddled me, saying "So strong!"). Mine was like any other childhood: a little awkward, a smidge insecure, and a tad meh. See, my personality, ever trusting, failed to see the shared circumstances and connections that my peers and I had. I was the ostracized chubbster, a loud kid stuffed inside a shy mind. It was my destiny, one that I was not accustomed to, and one that I fought with anger, fought with fists, fought with thoughts, and then ignored.

As the biggest kid in fourth grade, Tony knew his power, preying on the smaller to compensate for his gawkiness, and *this meant that I was his target. Day after day of inexcusable harassment and beatings in the recesses of the schoolyard, belittled and humiliated while being shoved into the girls bathroom and locked in for the entire recess. Choked against the wall on some days. Fear became anger, and anger became hate, and somewhere in there hate become a smattering of hope: suddenly, hoping that I wouldn't be noticed became the most important thing. I ducked in corners, quickly switching directions when his imposing frame revealed itself. As I lay there, tormented, my only respite became the better version of myself, a lucid dream amidst the beatings. I had avoided beatings for too long, living in shadows, and the hero that lay within me yearned to fight back. I was the Superman protector for those who couldn't speak for themselves. After all, that was the only measure a little boy could practice in dealing with the relentless nature of bullying.*

Like the hero's journey, my arch was imminent—seven years later, I was a far different figure than my youth, having bulked into the starting varsity fullback. The scars of my youth reverberated in my ferocious desire to succeed, and my periphery keenly observed those whose present paralleled my past. I wore an invisible "S" emblazoned on my chest, and my chance to soar to the aid of a peer came to fruition—my high school had a special education program for those with learning disabilities. One of our special needs students, Kyle, was being bullied by another student, who was forcing him to dig through trash and eat the half-eaten food that lay within. Other students gathered, laughed, jeered, or played ignorant and walked idly by.

Kyle, with his decreased ability to comprehend the sickening putrid prank, partook in the "joke," not realizing that the student body was laughing at him, not with him. Tap, tap. I fervently tapped on his shoulder in an effort to cease his unrecognized participation in the cruelty of the antic, then confronted the bully.

At first, I bulldozed him into the wall, and it took all of my willpower to keep from turning my fists into weapons. I breathed, the recesses of my past haunting my mind, and in a moment of calm, I chose to use words instead. If I persisted, I would be no better than Tony, who had choked my courage years ago. I knew empty threats had no impact on the bully, but the connection between Kyle and myself was clear—the ferocity that originated from the fury and frustration of my childhood had transformed into a virulent desire to help.

I walked away from the bully, grabbed Kyle's backpack from the ground, and guided Kyle back to his classroom. At the entrance, my words found their voice: "Kyle, you gotta stand up for yourself." I continued, lightheartedly: "If anyone messes with you again, send them my way!" In retrospect, I don't recall his reaction; it probably made very little difference, if any at all. I just needed to match the cadence of the scene, to attempt to heal a situation that would otherwise have remained warped.

And so I transport myself back to my new reality, Eve; unclench my tough love; and observe her needs. I see her hesitation, even from herself. Because there is an allure that radiates from Eve; ethereal, a vision of serenity that bathes and quiets the observer. Keen eyes and grace are embodied in a small, lithe frame. I sense something else in her enigmatic countenance: a quiet mix of ungrounded strength, a byproduct of age, life, and tenacity.

I take a step back, then another, then another, my vacillation of non-action matching hers. We step away from each other in tandem, until epiphany reaches us both. Eve is waiting for me to take the lead, and suddenly I'm ten years old again. My scrubs cover the "S" on my chest, and I waver in my touch. Her eyes grab my weakness.

In my mind, a thought began to pound one day, and then never stopped, pistons in my body like in a revving engine. Because that was the connection, and I missed it—I never picked up on my vibrating thoughts, instead anesthetizing them with distractions. Because bullying has that effect, detaching thoughts while they pulsate in your mind, and as you thud to the ground your feelings follow, numb and silenced. Scared and trembling, I learned to shut these down at first. Eve had shut these down, too, erasing the connection between that which hurt and that which injured. I needed to reach her before she fell to the proverbial ground, and this is where the transition occurred.

❖

She was active, a mover, shaking with nervous energy that was contained within her lithe frame. The complexity of physical control in martial arts was at her core—self-generated movements with reliance on the one and only iteration of self that she recognized.

The Doctor met her energy, recalcitrant, focused, keenly astute, and the symphony opened softly. It was a hint of harmony, as he probed toward the origin of her pain as it moved from part to part, quiet in its defiance, and she allowed it to travel, not yet trusting him. There was uncertainty: something was clearly going on, but the experts who should have been able to heal her came up empty. Treatment was a drug haze, but her eyes were too discriminating to allow it, a delicate power between strength and agility.

Like the Doctor, she had always been able to rely on her body to carry her through the tasks of her day, regardless of normalcy or extraordinary, all while keeping the self intact. Now her moments were filled with degrees of ache, hidden as the troubles of his youth; it was getting on their nerves now. And there was distraction: focus suffered—not at *the pain*, but at the why, the how, at "What can she do?" and "What *should* she do?"

There was disappointment: living day to day, but stuttered, so unlike her gliding frame. The strain became ceaseless, and each new movement produced a sting that she couldn't control. Each new ache instigated another to follow. This cycle was never-ending: hurt, injury, lack of conditioning, loss of strength, and then the fear of more injury.

There was martyrdom—this was her burden to carry, and the Doctor was shocked to see his own face in hers, a determination that derided help. The injury took form only when pushed, and hid so easily in the day-to-day that Eve barely let out a squeak. She was a silent soldier, and he knew, because he, too, had hidden the maladies in his thoughts and turned a smile to the world, but hope eluded him. Some days, she fought the temptation. Some days, she could barely hold the line. Some days, she lost.

On her first appointment with the Doctor, it was temptation that stymied her confidence—and she went to him, exasperated, because she first needed to exhaust her insured options. After a gamut of blood work, stress tests, and MRIs, she was declared to be in perfect health. Doctor after doctor, with the same facts and different notes, came to same conclusions despite taking various approaches. Yet the cost outweighed the cycle that had no end, and standard healthcare took a back seat. When she developed a bad spasm in her back, chiropractic care alleviated much of the neck and some of the back discomforts, but the benefits were temporary and didn't touch the headache or ribs or any of the other problems, which kept her near to square one. So she entered, hesitation on her end, amid a cacophony of interactions, silently anticipating the impending disappointment. He was unsure, awkward around her energy. Who was the lead? And so they danced, stepping on each other's toes.

❖

Knowing very well the biases in medicine when one sees much of their personal journey in their patient, the younger me had to evaporate. The "S" and the cape I had once loved wearing also had to be doffed. I donned my glasses and scrutinized, now a listener. Eve needed my hope now, and, as much as her journey called my lessons into action, I had to un-attach. I stepped back, avoiding toes, feeling, prodding, and—a-ha! A bundle of nerves, and a nerve root! A nerve bundle stuck out like a thorn in her stomach where the lumbosacral plexus formed, leading me to resistance—resistance that expanded to her coccyx (tailbone), which was bent. A nerve tension ran down her arms and legs, grappling onto every nook and cranny in her spine, head to toe.

Eve was armed with many protective layers, a cocoon of hidden weakness and strengths. I knew, and she knew that I hit something. I felt a shock and then quickly backed off, waiting to be invited in again.

Her world was tangled, like ivy that grew uncontrolled. It was unkempt. As a doctor, it was epic—I'd not yet felt anything so cluttered within. Like her, I also didn't have the absolute confidence in explaining the rationale behind her internal knots or her painful throbs. All I could do was walk with her on her journey.

I intended to be honest with Eve; I gave her my initial impression, yet disclaimed the possibility that perhaps the cause might be a shape-shifter. She stared at me, probing, and I pledged that I would find a remedy for this mess. Maybe it was the first genuine thing she had heard from someone in a medical position. Her eyes relaxed.

Each treatment was a step, one in which we had memorized the previous dance sequence and tepidly counted down, ready to work. She evolved, vacillating between relief, skepticism, interest, and determination. I listened, and I could almost hear her saying, "Finally, a doctor who listens!" The therapy wasn't traditional, and I had to reach deep into my toolkit, emerging with instruments I had studied but not used; desperate times called for desperate measures.

There was a string of concerns to address. A left wrist ache here, unstable ankles that strained easily there, a sunken rib, and headaches that matched her menstrual cycle. The only way to treat her was by being extended an invitation, and then

I progressed, softly placing pressure onto her abdomen. This is where I found the strand that led to her uterus as she rotated her neck. We began with visceral mobilization with her bladder and uterus, with her head turning from side to side. I moved to her ascending colon with functional movement patterns developed from the Institute of Physical Art (IPA). There are complex nerve bundles that traverse the course of visceral organs, directly or indirectly winding around the soft tissue that restrict mobility. This is what Eve needed to acquire, and it is what Jean-Pierre Barral, an osteopathic doctor in Europe, had developed.

I went there first, hoping Eve could experience my touch, and, although subtle, it resonated deep within her. Un-flexing her coccyx was my real goal, and, as explained by Gregory Johnson of the IPA, has many facets that need to be addressed. There are three possible factors that he believes benefit from IPA's Functional Mobilization Lower Quadrant™ courses.

1. *The nervous and connective tissue relationship attached to it are similar to the balloon holders at Disneyland, a single string with a hundred balloons. If he decides to change directions or turn his wrist in an awkward direction, the balloons above will follow suit; as one side rises up, the others will come down, a pendulum that requires balance. Lengthening the tension in our bodies, especially our nervous system, is instrumental to good health.*

2. *The biomechanical ramifications of a joint such as the coccyx needed to be taken into account, as it occupies an area like a thorn. When the pelvis and hip collide and inflame the nervous tissue, irritation is inevitable.*
3. *The connections to the pelvic floor and core muscles that facilitate motility of the colon and the length-tension to these muscles are vital to the physiological balance of the organs. I often observe patients that experience issues with their menstrual cycles or have incontinence of the bladder and/or bowel to have nerve root irritation.*

Buying into this complicated (yet infuriatingly simple!) origination of nerve root issues is often my biggest hurdle in healing for optimum health.

The explanations of her condition and how to address it were my main concern; I had to match her tempo of physiological knowledge, appealing to both her mind and her gut. At times, my explanations were lost on her, and her body contracted. As I learned to explain concepts as realities, so, too, did my understanding grow; we agreed that they resonated on a more intuitive, and perhaps even subjective component of my understanding.

This was where the dance started, as Eve began to lead, marking a shift from my three steps of healing: mobility, stability, and endurance. I had mobilized her body, stabilizing her mind, but her strength lacked a crucial component—her participation.

The truth is, my patients are the most integral part of their healing, and I can only lead my horse to water, so I armed her with plausible answers that satiated her brain. In actuality, this is what she craved the most: a harmony that resonated, notes that made sense, and treatments that seemed to be working.

Pain that was once limiting, edifying, and humbling were the keys to her treatment: limit the negatively suppressed thoughts, build upon a foundation of clarity and self-participation, and accept the reality as the origin to a brighter future. Hers was a challenge to overcome, a challenge that I, too, had to face after years in practice. Fighting the bully with hope—it worked.

❖

Her face revealed nothing, steadfast in her calm. She had the lucidity of awareness, recognition of where the pain lay, and how to put it to rest, a proper burial to the ebbing iteration of her previous self. She was involved. Right thought, right action—and she continued to glide through the movements without her partner. It was beautiful. She had chosen the path to heal, and lived each moment down to the very fiber of her nerves, for choices implied action and a willingness to work toward realizing a goal. Communication with the Doctor, dedication to her exercises, instilling new habits, and ceaselessly working to understand her triggers were key, as were building on an edifice that can endure the mental and physical fatigues of life.

And, like the pile of clutter that had once covered her mind, papers found files, pencils found holders, and wires were wrapped neatly. She practiced active participation—and she kept it up, trusting in her god, her faith, her knowledge that this, too, shall pass. And she passed, with the serenity and grace of her conviction. Hiding in clear sight, Eve learned to hope. Perhaps like the wind on a summer's eve, Eve's cape floats behind her, a hidden "S" on her chest.

❖

Rehab and Revive: A Practice is Born

Why does the body feel pain? Is it to cause us unnecessary stress? To immobilize our body and render it unusable for a period? Perhaps we consider injury as an unfair circumstance that mocks the ease of life. But perhaps there is a greater meaning to injury, and more—to the impact that it has on our lives. This vehicle in which we travel through life might create injuries as warning signs, entreating us to pay better attention or to slow down.

I can mention the physicality of injury—weakness, compensation, lack of awareness, overuse, and so on, but the salient truth is loud: our perception of immortality is pervasive, and by virtue we must work hard and play hard with a now-or-never mentality. We fear the silence of looking inward, rather busying ourselves with mindless chatter and movements. Everything is relative, and the world that is ceaselessly in competition cannot rest easy, so we become fierce, in both body and mind. And thus irresponsibility takes a shape.

Not too long ago, I was at the top of my game, a successful physical therapist in our nation's capitol, with fame to match, a physical powerhouse of ego. I suffered from a consistent lack of sleep, yet three hours of rest seemed sufficient for me to play on aggressive sports teams over the weekends, and I awoke frequently to play an early morning game of flag football.

One morning, three weeks after smashing my left ring finger and tearing a ligament, I experience pain after I foolishly played yet again. In hindsight, this small event was simply the precedent to an impending disaster, a warning call from my body to rest. This I ignored, masking the true issue with tape and continuing to play while it healed. Little did I know it was a small wave against the rising tide that was barreling my way.

Because this small injury wasn't big enough to get my attention, I forged ahead with even more vigor. Without even a second thought, I played on. As fate would have it, my first game went well, yet, without adequate pre-game warming exercise, my left knee felt slightly unstable, a bit askew. Within minutes of the second game starting, a sudden movement produced an audible *pop* and I fell. I almost instantly understood the cause of the injury.

Destiny and a torn ACL had me on the floor, finally demanding my full attention. Lamenting and loathing my fate, I cursed myself, yet rest coursed through my mind. Mine was a body without wheels, yet my car walked for me. A drive to the hospital produced a reckoning that this injury had not transpired in vain. Blowing through the first stop sign that the universe had provided me only accelerated my breakneck speed, yet I still couldn't connect the dots.

A torn ligament severed my connections to that fast-paced life, a social circle I couldn't run with anymore. Being bed-ridden for the weeks after surgery gave me the respite I needed, gave me time to rediscover, question, and quiet my mind. Agility replaced speed and awareness replaced the constant need, and I knew that my healing was ready to be shared. Packing my bags and returning home was my new relief, a respite that my mind demanded.

Coming home to Irvine, California, was symbolic—wide streets, "Children at Play" signs, and quiet shops. As my focus shifted, my vision cleared and I could see the forest despite the trees. Injury forced introspection, and, as my body healed, so, too, did my mind. Rehabilitating my mind had, in fact, revived my body, and my practice was born.

3

HEADSTRONG
Trust the Process

She rescheduled twice—called, scheduled, called, rescheduled, desperate for help, unable to find her footing. After too many doctors and too little to show for her efforts, physical therapy was a long shot, but the only one that didn't require *a* shot. It didn't require surgery, a scalpel, or a pill to numb her aches. Committing to the pain was just as confining as committing to another failed attempt. And still she rescheduled.

It was an evasion of sorts, her way of circumnavigating the tumultuous waters that she finally learned to swim parallel to, rather than against. She was, in essence, living with her injury, and it was a sad sight to see. Her surface bubbled confidently, full of nervous energy and disconnected movements and thoughts. Her patterns were evident in everything, especially as she walked, all parts moving independently of each other, brains in her feet, in her knees, in her hips—no connections anywhere. It was her foot that hurt, a toe that failed to yield, a random pain in her abdomen that didn't leave her.

"I can't bend it!" she exclaimed. "Is it because of my sesamoid fracture last year? I thought it would have healed by now!"

The Doctor leaned over her, squinting at her knees. "Let's see how you walk," he said. As he guided her to the hallway, keen eyes capturing every movement like frames of a picture, micro slices of a slow-motion reel, she walked—more like wobbled—through Therapy Room 1, Her legs whipping around, her short strides that didn't match her tall frame, and the constant shifting of her weight like a clock on speed were painful, for her both and the Doctor.

The side of her abdomen hurt. So did her back, on the same side as her unbendable toe—a connection in her disjointed body that made sense only to the Doctor, yet explanations would fall on deaf ears. She needed to feel it. And with long hair and purple tennis shoes, Ivy laid back, waiting for a miracle. That's what Yelp® told her to do. It was hard to follow the leader, but Ivy had penciled me in, ambiguous in her hope. Her wavering voice didn't match her absolute demand:

"I need my toe to move. And for some reason, my abdomen hurts. Isn't that strange?"

❖

Sitting back and observing, I'm faced with her constant twisting, popping, and stretching. Like a dancer, she's never still, a feisty fairy emerging from Never Never Land, never calm, never sure, constantly controlling. Not stable, not grounded, not silent. It's like I'm trying to catch a hummingbird. New thoughts blossom in my mind with her every step—unsteady, unstable. The body mirrors the mind, and I wondered, was it the chicken or the egg? Calmness leads to grounded results, while anxiety tends toward precarious conclusions. She wobbled around, and my eyes darted to follow her. A toe that didn't bend, an ankle that rolled, knees that buckled, thighs that remained steadfast, and a pelvis that seemed to dislike the rest of her body. Her voice was aggressive using medical terms: sesamoid, fifth-metatarsal surgery, plantar fasciitis, kidney this, intestinal that. Even I was exhausted by the litany, test after test to determine this or that. She was a problem analyst; everything short of perfection in her eminent mind was a failure.

Hers was a story akin to all who are incapable of fathoming failure; even careless injuries come as a shock. Her "Why me? This isn't fair! I have way too much to do to worry about this pain!" mentality typifies the societally successful (stressful?) healthcare consumer. I have encountered some patients whose all-encompassing need to micromanage the minutia of both themselves and their surroundings are often the least-prepared for the healing process. The irony is not lost on me because a humble mind is the gateway to truly mending, and, despite their perfectionist tendencies, the ego of ignoring the pain becomes the largest stumbling block. Because of that mentality, attaching themselves to a diagnosis or disorder is the only "logical" explanation to a limited world and belief system; it becomes something to blame.

In fact, this avoidance is so dominant in their behavior that it eventually comes to dominate their mind. It defines them. The label of "injury" gives them the right to blame the external world, sustaining their belief in the rightness of a reality in which their diagnosis is not married to their actions, allowing them to blame an unfair atmosphere. These types of patients hold so desperately to these logical explanations that they become paralyzed, despite the severity (or lack) of their malady. The result is extreme, two ends of a divergent spectrum: half completely melt down, too fearful, too vigilant, and too afraid, resigning themselves to the injury as their new reality, confined by the label, while the others live in complete denial and continue to ignore the affliction. The powerful feedback loop that dominates their mindsets—avoiding pain, defined by pain, scared of *pain, avoiding pain—is extremely difficult to treat, because the rehabilitation of the mind is far more important than physical manipulations. The fear of the unknown lies in their minds, and this mental chatter causes more harm than any physical activity. Challenging their preconceived notions is key to shifting their paradigms of thought.*

One more couldn't hurt, and I matched her tone. "Stand up, and don't let me push you down." Her knees buckled under my slight push, and she seemed confused and shocked at her own weakness. Maybe this was the beginning of a new reality in which disability was the impetus to seek me out.

"But I did Crossfit...I'm in great shape," she protested. "Actually, that's the reason that I broke my toe—it happened during my workouts, and I haven't really been able to walk properly since."

Coming to terms is such an exhausting process. I can relate to the days of "no pain, no gain" and "stronger, faster, harder"—everything short of working out to the point of collapse was a frivolous regimen in life. Breaking a toe was simply a small tragedy in mind over matter; broken hearts and broken feet were all a failure in educating the true necessity of balance, silence, and moderation.

Her symptoms had been confused with their roots, a connection that she couldn't see or feel, but was obvious to me. Her pelvis had divorced itself from her hip, which had fought with her knee, which was not speaking to her ankle. The result? Her feet received messages from no one, a supply chain broken by a lack of communication that regarded no one as a leader.

Even as the leader of my own body, my high school injuries seemed absolutely divergent from my late-twenties aches and pains, which ultimately seemed unlinked to my early-thirties heart issues. Here a pain, there a pain—I called it sports injury, a lack of balance, a bad knee, or age. Doctors who specialized in these maladies assigned them this treatment, or that, separate pills for separate pains, and root after root was ignored, while symptom after symptom was celebrated. I call these migrating miseries: a game of whack-a-mole ensues in our culture when one injury is smashed (either "healed" surgically or masked with pills) and another magically appears elsewhere. No medical textbook teaches us to observe and analyze the totality of the picture, to see the forest despite the trees, to connect the dots and draw a conclusion.

In my case, they drew blood. Blood tests, MRIs, CAT scans, and bone density exams were performed, all with singular results: localized injuries caused by singular events, and this pill or that tendon removal would do the trick. And it did—until it didn't. It was only when I began truly to absorb the lessons brought to me that I furthered my horizon line; I needed to find a reason for why my body was not efficient or healthy, instead of just bandaging a wound that was too deep to heal.

The body, I learned, wants to be healthy: we have the most brilliant cleansing digestive and mobility system that we have studied, something that science is unable to replicate. Our original parts perform in an entirely different league than do artificial replacements. We are built for success, Spartans with the innate potential for absolute agility and strength. Our mind creates chasms of patterns that pull our bodies along for the ride. We fall into failure because the squeaky wheel gets the grease, and we ignore signs until the pain starts. In our society, we ignore our natural bodies from birth, filling up our blood with formulas, sitting instead of standing, eating instead of exercising. Why? Because our medical system encourages us to stay unhealthy, because treating a chronic and preventable condition (like obesity, heart disease, or asthma, the biggest killers in America) is much more profitable than preventing it. We cure, but we don't prevent. We treat the pain, not the cause. We use too much because it costs so little. But the cost is very high, to both our bodies and our wallets. This disconnection between how we move and feel is severed, because the extremely negative physical results are easily masked by surgeries and medications that are designed to keep us healthy enough to keep abusing and utilizing the system. No one wants to be treated—they want to be tended to. They want to be passive instead of being assertive.

So I tend to her, knowing that the root will eventually reveal itself. Ivy, on her back, her mind in one place and her body in another, exists as the epitome of the American medical consumer, and she can't walk because of it. I pull on her toe; no reaction. I push on her toe; no reaction. With my tool that I frequently use to aid in breaking up connective tissue that hinders smooth movement, I slowly begin to free up her surface restrictions, the only connected parts of her body—her tendons, which have fused themselves to her soft tissue, forcing her toes to remain frigid and distorted. Perhaps it was the years of heels, or perhaps it was genetics, she muses, maybe it was even the injury a few months ago! But I know this not to be true, and soon enough, I won't be able to shield the reveal. Because everything is linked—our bodies are blocks of power that diffuse from one to the next. I find the tendon, take a deep breath that I tell her to share with me, and set it free. The anxious energy seems to hang in silence for but a moment, a chill in the California air, and then the release sets in. She is my loudest patient.

❖

"Oh my God!" her voice echoes throughout the office. "Stop hurting me!" The Doctor smiles for the future, because the question is coming: "Can you bend your toe?" He wants to ask if a sufficient miracle was performed, but the answer is there: it moves. Just a wiggle, a slight bend, and a yelp of joy, because she believes that she's healed, that her foot is now able again, and that her heels and hikes await her. The Doctor continues, because symptoms aren't roots, and roots feed the body. She stands, knees over toes, a spring to her step. There were no more excuses in her way, and this sudden about-face was absorbed into her psyche as quickly as her prior resignation to her random pains. Everything in her was a series of impulsive arbitrations that she formed in her mind—"I'm perfect! I'm broken! I'm healed!"—so once was enough.

But the problem remains: only part of her is healed. The others are again ignored and forgotten, a body that her mind as broken into segments. She could only see the iceberg for the tip, not wanting to know what lay beneath the layers of her body or the years of her mindset. After her session, the Doctor ventured deeper, because he recognized avoidance—in fact, he invented avoidance; glossing over problems meant that he was in control: study harder, work out harder, think harder, until it becomes harder to live. Not wanting to accept her reality, Ivy settled for an iteration in which his words fueled her defiance against introspection, and the disconnection reached her mind.

Three months of here and there, and she drops by in lax commitment, elated at the results, a ballerina with a twist. Because, although the mechanics have healed, no longer disjointed gears to no end, her body still aches. There is no respite from herself, and by continuously ignoring the origins of her pain, her healing is superficial. Her abdomen and back still cause her pain, yet she is unable to see the correlation, because we aren't taught to see the links, because we're discouraged from seeing too much and learning too much and being too much a part of ourselves.

Severing the habits of the mind is the third step in the healing process, because mobility, strengthening, and endurance (self-sufficiency in the mind and self-empowerment of the body) are the only routes of significance. She refuses to truly commit, to participate in the possibility of her body, and her disengagement overshadows her frame. Her mind is quick to absorb the changes that will make its route easier, though, and her biomechanics reflects that shift.

Month three, and her gait is perfect. Her agility is obvious and her strength comes through in waves. But her pain hasn't lessened. It's hidden within her frame, a pulsing organ that yells louder than she does. Her visceral ache originates between her fear and her hope, the root of all her maladies. Her nerve root is to blame.

❖

The excess chatter quieted, the stretching paused, and a wide-eyed look came from Ivy. I know I touched a nerve this time; Ivy is silent. She doesn't trust the process, and, just like the source of her pain, it's a topic she wants to ignore. "Why don't the exercises heal me?" she asks repeatedly, avoiding my gaze, avoiding her own. I've been there, though, bypassing until I was boxed into a corner. My scars are proof enough that I picked at it until I ran out of options, with my only recourse being acceptance of my issue. Acceptance is not resignation; it is the opening note to life's symphony—empowerment. My only choice was to let it be, and that required as much active participation as I could muster. But with Ivy, the fear lies deeper, because I'm her last hope. And so I begin to dissect, probing, reticent, matching responses with motion.

There's no more room in her mind for limitations, and just as I removed the fascia that bound toe to tendon, I must separate organ from nerve. It is excruciating—not for her body, but for her mind, tearing away the layers of doubt that confine her, destabilizing the nerves that aided in her prison, lengthening the L5–S1 nerve root from its compression. Because I know one thing: her lower back and abdomen pain are the cause of her foot pain. The lumbosacral plexus nerve bundle that rests in her pelvic region had an omnipotent presence throughout her body, and, as the mechanics of her frame healed, the nerves that had remained dormant were now sparked to life, desperately attempting to subvert and distract. Her nerve issue was biomechanically anchored, but *a product more of her mental anxiety at the loss of options. Solving that was the key to her freedom, and so I began the final phase of treatment.*

I pressed on organs, feeling my way through the internal muck, experiencing her history from her body, my fingers relaying a common occurrence. We were both forced to overcome the monsters in our minds that had personified themselves in pinched nerves and tight tendons. She cried out, not from discomfort, but from confusion, desperately holding on to her last notion of what was and the fall into the beginning of what would be. It was tedious and frustrating for us both, but the line was blurring; was this the past or the future that was holding her back?

Freeing her scar tissue and providing her mobility sat well on the surface, but even that failed to change her perspective, because to Ivy, perfection was the goal. And despite the lifetime of compartmentalizing aches, her excuses didn't match up. The seed had been planted in her first visit: "We need to go further," the Doctor had said. "The origin is not what you think." It grew quietly within her brain, illuminating the blocks of connections that traveled throughout her body, and finally readied her for a change. I performed one final manipulation, this one more visceral than the rest, and she lay still, drained, numb, and resigned. I waited for the inevitable as something activated. Perhaps it was herself. She felt a tingle.

❖

Tingles of hope relayed to her toes and obliterated worry, aligned with newfound movement. She felt normal but not, ready but unprepared, informed but confused. Because now all hope was exhausted, and all options seemed spent. The release came in oscillations of prickles of feeling, but the Doctor knew why. He had released her from the restraints, a revitalization that started in the mind and rehabilitated the body. It required one final yet critical part of the equation—her.

As her body altered, her mind remained steadfast, or so she thought. Unbeknownst to her, the metamorphosis emanated from the top down, a trickledown that sparked each synapse as it traveled, freeing her knees, her toes, her brains, her habits. And without knowing, the belief was unbelievable.

Thus, hers was a timid involvement and elicited a timid reaction. There was no more Doctor, no more tape, no more excuses. Indeed, the lonely road of repression from her earned injuries now came to a fork. It was the juncture of earned versus learned behavior, as her hip needed this thrust at that angle that originated from that thought and this knowledge.

She was now armed with daily exercises with names that echoed titles in the comedy of the absurd (Ballerina! Buttwalking! Pinch Push Pinch!). "No more stinking thinking!" he reminded with a smile. "Work through your fear. It's all in your mind." She had reached the apex of the shift, and her invigorated nerves pulsated in their newly released intensity.

Tingles turned into connections, connections into building blocks of power that transferred from her un-aching side to her bendable toe, and blocks of power into clarity of mind. Just like correct walking patterns helped her biomechanics, so, too, did amended thoughts aid in the healing of her negative thought patterns that elicited the plethora of her symptoms. Just like the Doctor predicted (or created), diffusion took its course. Fear was the pain, pain was the band-aid, band-aids were excuses, and excuses were fear. She felt no more fear as she ventured into the unknown. It was a small step for her foot, a giant leap for herself. Ivy walked on.

4

SHORTCUTS
The Case for Prevention

Retrospection is the universal human yearning in which hindsight is 20/20 and the mistakes of elapsed ages are lessons learned. But applying them again is impossible, and so we move ever-fervently forward, hoping that the future is not dictated by our former selves, but rather that it is shaped by them. But that's the rub: can we talk to our old selves, warn them of their impending mistakes, and apply the Grandfather Paradox? If we go back and change the past, will we even be around in the present, hoping against hope that our fate will be our own?

Jed, 13 at the time, unaware of the consequences of poor athletic training, poor stretching habits, and years of ignorant wear and tear on his body, was an unexpected chance at personal redemption. Finally, an opportunity to prevent my inevitable pain! He was young, serious, and insecure, a byproduct of weight that he carried both in his heart and on his frame. He trusted no peer, instead distancing himself from the chronic solitude that eventually defined him. Before his injury occurred, an intervention to break his shell was needed. Alice, his mother, full of the wisdom needed to learn from observation rather than experience, was the vehicle to time-travel against the ache.

It has often been said that we grow up trying to solve problems that we couldn't remedy in our youth. Jed—quiet, too old for his years—was the proof that time travel was possible. He was the Doctor's salvation.

❖

An interesting thing goes on in the therapy room. It's like a time capsule stalled in age and space. Therapists can facilitate redemption, and it often comes in the form of this patient with that ache and that patient with this pain, yet rarely are we presented with the prospect of total preventative care. Perhaps, at times, healers themselves are desperate to believe in something magical to restore others so that they can secretly hold onto the possibility of restoring themselves—a better version of ourselves, if you will. Perhaps we're all looking for validation of some sorts. This would be mine.

Alice, Jed's doting mother, was herself a prior patient of mine; she'd had a series of pains that culminated in a snapping of her lower back after a bout with pneumonia. Daunting, distracting, frustrating—these were our shared feelings, as victims of learned traits and jarring physical habits. There was no guidebook on correct patterns of movement; our society is inundated with quick fixes that yielded no lasting carryover, full of doctors that are held captives by their syringes and scalpels, spreading sensational truths on how to lose weight and exercise, creating the picture of optimal health.

Her story wasn't news to me, just to a plethora of too many people with too many preventable problems: a snap in her lower back caused her to knees to buckle; a pain that radiated ferociously down her neck, back, arms, and legs; and a feeling of being broken. Adding insult to injury, a car accident put her back into a state of constant pain, reduced her functionality, and caused her depression. The result? Opting out of activities that made her feel useless, weak, sad, and scared.

It was all avoidable, and that's what frustrated me, because an ounce of prevention is worth a pound of cure. Alice learned this the hard way, as her life was limited from the harmony of opera to the cacophony of giving up after the first act. We spent months tracing the symptoms to the source, and—slowly—the *signs revealed themselves: poor posture led to poor respiratory circulation, resulting in pneumonia, which culminated in a weaker back, and snap! Alice began to amend from the inside out. To her, it was challenging, educational, and rewarding. And, like myself, her healing meant sharing, transferring the wisdom of observing and learning.*

I met Jed, and I was transported to my 13-year-old self, a chubby and nervous teen who was too eager to prove himself. I knew what lay in his future: an athletic career that dominated his mind, a ferocious attachment to achieving the perfect human form, and, ultimately, injuries that would render him incapable of living a fully physically optimal life. Eager, excited, and enlightened, I was ready to mold Jed into the man I yearned to have been, without wasted years learning from injuries that limited my very self. That, too, was a fallacy that I had to transform, because it was a catch-22: without the aches of my youth, I would have been unequipped to motivate and facilitate others, and so this was my vicarious hope coming to life. I began at the beginning and looked into my past.

❖

This was not treatment; rather, it was a defensive play that the Doctor had spent years preparing for after a lifetime of offensive injuries. They met on neutral ground—a local field near his house that demonstrated not his inefficiencies, but his capabilities. The Doctor watched, his youth before his eyes, and began to see the body for its parts: blocks of movement and muscle that were seemingly untainted. A sudden movement and he was reminded of his shoulder injury, another twist and his broken leg floated into his consciousness. A diagnosis: initially, he was predisposed to a weaker left side and nerve tension that inclined him toward imminent injuries. The geometry of his body had not revealed its weaknesses, but the keen eyes of the Doctor sifted through the matrix of physical information.

Silent, insecure, jaded, with clunky movements to match a chaotic mind, Jed exuberated a singular flaw—a disconnect between what his body was and what his mind imagined it to be. He was a cadet, empathetic to the plights of others, but distanced, an observer of a kind. He had decent potential but a weak core, poor posture, and an itch to rapidly build muscle, like every hormonal teenage boy. They oscillated between building foundations that were anchored to all parts of his body while simultaneously correcting habits. That resolution leads to the rebuilding of the developmental sequence—proper rolling, crawling standing, sitting, walking, and running form. "Wax on, wax off!"—it was a monotonous routine of repetition, training, mobilizing, and endurance. Jed wanted more, part of the youthful desire to be faster and stronger, competing against his friends who were rapidly gaining weight and strength, and he wondered why he was stuck with rolling and crawling activities. But the Doctor knew, imparting the process, testing Jed's patience and hunger like a drill sergeant ingraining in his recruits the smallest of details: education on biomechanics and lessons on awareness. Building the intention for consciousness of every detail was critical; ignoring even minor details would be a pivotal mistake, because "masters do the basics well" (Jeff Ellis, 2012, p. 34, *FMT Foundations*).

The goal was simple: solidify the foundation of mindful movement, arrange the body to absorb growth and motion, and then allow it to organically build strength and correct form. But for the Doctor, the abstract methods of correcting, repairing, healing, and fixing were not in his tool belt; averting danger instead of reeling from it was the new treatment plan. It was an unyielding opportunity to put into action what was merely a thought—squashing the pain before it began was possible.

The medical profession does less to preclude ailments than to treat them. It has been said that insurance companies would rather foot the bill of surgery because doing so is cheaper than preventing someone from having surgery. This is due mainly to the fact that prevention for the masses is far more expensive than paying for the occasional treatment or surgery every so often. Even that logic is flawed because the rates of chronic injuries and illnesses are rising, further straining the wallets of Americans. The business model encourages poor health.

This pervasive mentality is a major component that dictates the current state of our society—chronically pained, typically unhealthy, and in dire need of constant care. This is the crux of the issue as the medical industry continues along a treatment-first philosophy, because the less we participate in nipping our habits in the bud, the more reliant we become on relentless care. Solutions-based medicine and self-empowerment are divorced from the equation. The Doctor and his patients had been ingrained into that omnipresent mentality. True patient- and person-first healing, like injury, had to originate internally, as part of a concerted effort to actively make healthy choices through a healthy mind.

❖

Eight months of grueling training were required for both his mental and physical cores. For the same reason that military cadets are diligently trained in the proper mechanisms of firearm operation before they're ever handed a real weapon, Jed had to master his body before training at the gym. The process, however frustrating, was my prospect at deterrence. Because I, too, was in a race with myself, against a youth spent competing without thinking.

Watching the guy next to him at the gym would ruin him. Taking lessons from the seemingly athletic kid in school would crush him. Being a guy that he thought he ought to be at the gym would rob him of a life free of injury. The intention to notice is the mindset that needs to invade our nation, because, whether the injury that my patients, like so many, face is based upon earned or inherited circumstances is inconsequential. It is crucial to our treatment, and—more importantly—the avoidance of our injuries requires that we perform all our physical actions with a focused and clear mind. Jed was the embodiment of this notion, and it was my duty to ceaselessly impart his duty to his self.

Imparting advice sounds easy, and, just like the story of foolishness, we must all learn from experience. I, too, had fallen into that trap; my initial experiences as a physical therapist were full of more vigorous and emphatic application of knowledge of the how than a true tactile understanding of the whys. This lead to a series of popping backs and forced, high-velocity manipulations and applying "cool" techniques before I fully understood the safety and screening of truly rehabilitating: the true power of manipulations. To exercise the proper power, I needed to get back to the basics, committing myself to extra learning and studying for the coveted Certified Functional Manual Therapy title to be one of only a select population of Functional Manual Therapists. These studies forced me to revisit fundamental principles of movement and anatomy that humbled my fast-paced mind. I discovered that only using trendy techniques without the correct guidance as to when and why cheated my patients of the true art of fixing the body. I was no better than a technician, and I didn't value the true responsibilities of being a skilled, licensed healthcare professional. I learned the ABCs so I could write the story of wellness. Jed, like most adolescents, had to master the basics first, and that's where we began.

❖

Fourteen-year-old Jed was rushed into the Doctor's office with swollen legs and a bruised ego, because trusting in the process meant adhering to the pace, and Jed had decided that a run on the beach was well deserved. Forgetting form and function, he continued—two miles, five miles, ten miles, exacerbating an injury and ignoring the pain. This was the derivation, that pain wasn't strength, that working through the aches didn't amount to working harder, and that big muscles aren't necessarily stalwart. The diagnosis was shin splints.

A frantic wakeup call roused the Doctor, too, but training ensured that he saw through the symptom to the core, and his attention was vital. It wasn't shin splints, but an inflamed anterior compartment, and it seemed to be getting a worse. This concern was not to be taken lightly, and he considered calling an ambulance and trying to use manual therapy to help reduce the pressure on the blood vessels, nerves, and muscles. Research has shown that the only way to help compartment syndrome of the legs was surgery, while it has not been proven that loosening the fascia would have a verifiable impact. But this was when challenge met opportunity; as the voice of his educators echoed, possibilities abound. The Doctor remembered this, his mind inching toward cautious resolution while his fingers geared toward defiant movement.

Fortunately, the swelling reduced with every stroke of his palm—up toward the lymphatic system (the sewage system of the body), back down in therapeutic massage. He used a rubber plunger that mimicked the ancient oriental medicinal technique of cupping. Tension eased into hope. With Jed looking on nervously, the Doctor, reticent for the greater part of half an hour, finally opened his mouth, exhaling the trepidation that had filled his mind. What escaped in words was admonishment to Jed to make mindful decisions, follow the rhythm of his body, and never let his ego override his mind again.

These learned were lessons in concert with one another, relaying them to overarching habits in attentiveness to action. A setback that was caught early and repaired proved the process. Injury can be avoided and, if caught early, can be nothing more than a lesson learned. After a lifetime of physical and mental struggles, the value was priceless to the Doctor, as a new cycle revealed itself: awareness, empowerment, and endurance, a process designed to protect, and Jed was sold.

Now 16, strapping, and secure, Jed was the epitome of health, pursuing more than just heavy weights. He was the vicarious vehicle of optimum strength, absolute awareness, and perfect prevention, and the Doctor beamed. With inner strength, muscles didn't matter, only supplementing a life lived with intention. Here was a life that learned from observation, with wisdom at the onset, following a path of least resistance. Whether creating it or traveling it didn't matter, because the cycle was continuous. A cycle has many elements, often broken down into an infinite series of parts, each building upon the last, and yet all work toward the same end. Whether it was a lesson in experience or observation, the conclusion was the same: control the mind, control the body. Jed, through the stages, mirrored the Doctor, and shone like a reflection.

5

CHOOSE LIFE
Leaving the Cycle of Pain

"Give me a color," commanded the mentor. "Describe to me how it looks when your pain starts."

Quivering in hesitation, Dr. Lin inhaled in short spurts. "Black...it feels..." He paused before resuming speaking. "It feels like there's a black hand over my heart. I feel weak." The words escaped, finding refuge in the Doctor's mentor, Gregg. Fragility was met with Gregg's steady hands, steady gaze, and steady intuition. Vulnerable on the treatment table, his once-tanned skin was now a pallid white; he lay motionless, fully surrendered to the mentor, the visionary, and the juxtaposition between therapist and student was evident. Unadorned by labels, ego, or garb, the transition from Doctor to Justin was more than symbolic; it was vital. No longer could Justin hide behind the fears masked by his accolades and titles. Nor did Gregg care for these; he was more intrigued by the challenge of a critical moment. Pauses were met with resoluteness, fear with audacity, and novice-ness with mastery.

His classmates watched with bated breath, mirrors of his patients, with big eyes and gaping mouths, at the finesse of their mentor, Gregg Johnson, sachem of the healing arts in Functional Manual Therapy. Justin was his student, yet a leader to some, who offered his aches and pains for remedy, although the pressure was the origin. Too high, too sudden, too much, the pressure pulsed through his heart, and he was a victim of something that is all too common in an overworked culture.

Due to severe Stage 2 hypertension, Justin Lin had been prescribed 500 mg of Lisinopril, which he was to take twice a day, forever. But wait, that's not all! Zoloft to treat the resulting anxiety, and a bottle to numb the pain—was it twice a day? Four? Once? It didn't really matter how many times—it was enough. It was a dosage he couldn't digest, yet he mentioned it in passing in his encounter with Gregg.

The labels slowly came off with the outer clothing; layers of schooling and ego evaporated before the class, emerging as time ticked backward, exposing Justin. On the treatment table, there was nowhere to hide, and his tension screamed. Gregg possessed an awareness of movement and signals that transcended the senses, and there was no divergence from root to symptom. There was a void in the room, a quietness that seemed unnatural in its inherent existence, and it remained unnamed. As the fear in Justin's eyes was laid bare, the void found a title: fearless. This was the mentor, a man committed despite the possibility of failure, only because the possibility of success existed simultaneously.

Black was a color that encompassed his fear, the derivation of a pain that originated from years of control, from muddy attempts at achieving what only time could grant him: absolute calm in observation in healing. So the therapy began, the pain of facing his encumbrances surfaced, and it was suddenly too much pressure to handle. Gregg placed a firm hand on his carotid pulse—a vague diffused beat to the left side—and then looked away, feeling, sensing, and absorbing. There's something strange that happens to nerves of the autonomic system that don't glide past the muscles of the neck. The Phrenic nerve provides signals to our major life sustaining muscles, most importantly the diaphragm. The diaphragm affects our organs and strength to our core muscles of the trunk. The Vagus nerve affects all our organs and too much excitement of this nerve elicits feelings of stress from the mind to the body. This cranial nerve that originates from the brain, weaving through the body and finally reaching the bladder and sex organs affects the totality of our being.

He mobilized branches of the Phrenic and Vagus nerve, but felt no movement. A lack of flexibility created a void of constriction. Justin's fear froze his freedom.

❖

My name is Gregg, and I believe that I'm a student of the art of healing, of motion, of function, and a facilitator of mobility. I recall our first interaction; an overconfident email five years ago came from a boisterous D.C. physical therapist whose reputation preceded him, Dr. Justin Lin. There was urgency in his nonchalant queries, though, a desire to further his healing prowess by learning the art of Functional Manual Therapy, a form of physical therapy that advanced touching into transforming via the science adapted from my time at Kaiser Vallejo. This is where I spent countless years learning physical therapy and a form of neurological rehabilitation from my mentor, Maggie Knott. It was her and Dr. Herman Kabat's vision in the mid-1940s to develop a method of therapy that they called proprioceptive neuromuscular facilitation (PNF) after being commissioned by Henry Kaiser's son, who had multiple scleroses.

PNF—coupled with my teachings from Moshe Feldenkrais' Awareness Through Movement and many of the great manual therapists, including Rolfers, Trigger Point, and massage therapists of the time—led me to create my first soft tissue mobilization class in the 1970s. Functional Manual Therapy was born sometime thereafter as a hybrid of all these effective methods, with its roots still based on PNF.

Our first meeting was in a formal classroom setting, and his veneer of title, education, ego, and broken parts all glued together was transparent to my gaze; I had learned long ago to see the forest despite the trees—and now, how to sculpt trees to add to the forest. I approached his traits one by one, demolishing them, forcing him to rebuild his sense of self to rise above the motions. My candor may be daunting to some, yet his foundation was strong, including the code of ethics that resonated with his oath, and a voracious desire to learn how to observe not from learned text, but from earned touch.

This is how I vet the future of our field. Are you an oracle of optimizing health, not on the surface but in the core, posterior, anterior, coccyx, lumbar, organ, mind, heart, intention? Above all, shying away from certainty and moving toward possibility was the true transitional shift, because it is the constancy of awareness that leads to hacking away at the inessentials.

He was wearing too many hats, holding too many titles, and bearing too many pressures. His was a burden that transcended his primordial ego, reaching his mind and stressing his heart, as is the nature of it. Justin lived against his own grain, and, despite helping his patients with a ferocity of knowledge, a disconnect between intention and attachments to effectiveness was his Achilles heel. Invincibility is the most obvious sign of weakness; a hole in the shield is often more detrimental than no protection at all, only because it lures us into a false sense of security. His impenetrable facade had cavities deep enough to let the pain through, and he needed a manipulation of mind and spirit to heal those he so desperately sought to transform.

His heart was an unusual case, and rarely would someone seek the care of a physical therapist to resolve high blood pressure, so this was no ordinary opportunity. Patients do not surprise me much anymore, but I continue to be intrigued. It was critical to treat.

I pressed; there was a lack of Phrenic and Vagus nerve mobility, and a dearth of flexibility or a restriction may create unnecessary compression. This in turn falsely alarms the fight-or-flight autonomic nervous system, creating a perception of stress and heightened blood pressure that typically gets the body ready for action. The most negative impact is that this chronic inflammation (essentially a constant state of alarm in the body) breaks down healthy tissues, including those of an overworked heart. In Justin's case, it was an overworked mind that needed genuine healing. And it was at this juncture that spoke to me.

Rehabilitating his spirit was the key to reviving his mind, which would then be the formula to mending his body—and Justin was itching for a cure.

❖

Pills. It was a future that many succumb to, yet few desire, particularly Justin. This was an assault on more than his body; it drilled through the very core of his identity as a professional. Relying on external forms of healing was not his strong suit, especially after years of touting personal responsibility. And this was where the identity of knowledge, education, and title became burdens; it was the transformative shift between realizing that the pill was a crutch, and the therapy was the door to unlocking himself. Opening the door to self-reflection is impossible without a firm commitment, and that often cannot be garnered until desperation meets resolve. For Justin, this was the essence of his choice to practice Functional Manual Therapy, hence his need to trust in his mentor, the only one whose ability to see through the pain was by virtue, allowing patients to overcome it.

When bodies break, people become inherently selfish, pulling them into the prison of fear and limitations, victims of their own pain. It is the most personal of journeys; they are utterly alone, entirely lonely, enclosed in a windowless room away from a detached society. Distortions and contortions of a disconnected mind, body, senses, and intentions consume those just hoping to survive. In his experience, this was the most universal of sentiments of those with unresolved pain.

Rational thinking was not available. He feared reprisals from his peers, along with the possibility that perhaps the perception of Justin that he had so long portrayed—confident, bombastic, unbreakable—would be shattered, and he contracted under the pressure. The feelings of guilt and shame that were rooted in him now revealed his weakness, vulnerability, and, ultimately, his facade. Worst of all, he felt wholly responsible, with no crutch on which to lean. But that wasn't the case; he was the epitome of physical perfection, with a rigorous exercise schedule. Medical research dictating that he lose 10 pounds to lower his blood pressure resulted in his immediate action. Altering his diet changed the trajectory of his health. He smiled through the fear, yet the pressure remained.

❖

I have an interesting perception of failure. It is purely sensational, an amalgamation of fear and insecurity that binds us to an inevitable mindset. Justin did everything he needed (or so he thought) to lower his blood pressure, yet the numbers didn't add up, and the situation was becoming increasingly tense and precarious. Even a doctorate in DPT couldn't shield someone like Justin from himself, and I could feel the question gnawing at him: "Why heal others when I can't even heal myself?"

A commitment to the question was what overtook Justin's mind, but after years of observation, the real question hung in the air: "Will the cycle of my pain ever stop?" It was this worry that constricted his view, his mind, and his arteries. It isn't as though the fear rooted itself irrationally, because it was more a failure of the heart that Justin was succumbing to. He was struggling with a loss of hope, and suddenly I was his last option.

I was a witness to his evolution, a haphazard patchwork life filled with a cycle of injuries and surgeries, band-aids that held for a short period and then unraveled. Put back together, threaded, revived, over and over as his injuries mounted, each more debilitating than the last. His last injury was a severe insult, an assault on perseverance that killed his last chance for the eternal hope that Justin embodied for his patients. "What about the possibility I sold to my patients?" I heard him mull to himself. "Maybe there were no possibilities, no options, no choice." The thought loomed in his depressed mind, a destiny of demise, a letdown of epic proportions to his ego and his identity. As mind fell, so followed his body, and increasing pressure choked his already shortened breath. More than anything, illuminating the fact his asking "Why me?" was the cause of his continued suffering was indispensable to changing his outlook. And only his outlook would alter his vision and, subsequently, his heart.

I pressed firmly against his sternum and rib cage, guiding his breath to his heart, to his core, to his mind, tearing away the labels that restricted his heart and lungs. The heat under my hand ensured that the pressure was the appropriate amount. This "fascial burn" was akin to lava to his being. He shook, a violent spasm of fear leaving the body, welding joints to thoughts, regenerating movement more in the heart than in the body. His life-sustaining breath and heartbeat were restored.

Qualities were made into quantities, but a singular focus illuminated my periphery, overtaking my vision, guiding my hands along his body, transferring observation into experience in a shift that occurred from my fingertips to his brain. Justin breathed purposefully, inhaling the totality of the encounter with a sanguine expectation that his spirit would be restored.

Commit to a goal and don't waver, come what may. Justin had a crisis of identity and one of faith, and restoration was key. His last hope should have been his first choice, but all's well that ends well. A crisis of faith is what leads to a crisis of failure, which leads to a crisis of life, and we cannot divorce the brain from the body. Getting up slowly, Justin found his legs, felt his heart, gathered up his pieces, and took stock of himself. I *observed from a distance, inhaling with him until the pressure was off.*

❖

His legs swung over the therapy table. Justin found his footing slowly, availing himself of his choice to live with freedom, replete with endless possibilities to pursue. Gregg smiled as Justin met him in a grateful embrace, leaning over and whispering into Justin's ear. Relief and a smile resulted from this secret between two men, a challenge to heal with purity of thought and intention. Classmates continued to observe; the fourth wall was broken again, and a tender moment was shared by all. *Control-Alt-Delete*—the old labels he couldn't swallow were replaced with certainty, and so were the pills. Justin's pulse beat strong.

❖

Resolve met intention, and Justin went home, checking his schedule: Monday 10:45am – Lucas: my former coach's son, the one with cerebral palsy; a new patient whose case is intriguing even in theory. But the secret between he and his mentor resonated in his mind, pulsed through his body, and beat through his brain, because it was a prescription that went down smoothly.

Injuries arise, pain exists, and challenges burden. Survival is inherent, but thriving is more than a provocation of muscle; it is a core choice that is birthed from the mind, inaugurating the first step, unmasking the heroism of empowerment. The cloak was removed.

Choose life.

CANDID

An Interview with Gregg Johnson, Co-Founder of the Institute of Physical Art

What was the impetus for your pursuit and creation of Functional Manual Therapy (FMT)?

In my early years, my primary focus was to become the best PT possible. I do not remember envisioning developing a new system of manual therapy. I just had a desire to help people overcome their symptoms and enhance their function. Understanding optimal human function has always been a fascination. Probably the most pivotal component of my early professional experience was being blessed to spend seven years working with Maggie Knott at Kaiser Rehabilitation Center in Vallejo, California. The brilliance of the PNF approach offered me a platform to develop my skills. The tools of PNF offered me a system through which I effectively enhanced my patient's neuromuscular function and motor control. These skills provided me the confidence to offer hope to patients with any diagnosis. During these formative years at Kaiser, it became obvious to me that mechanical dysfunctions of the soft tissue and the articular systems were major factors limiting my neurological and orthopedic patients' progress. As a result of this insight, I began developing our soft tissue mobilization approach to address the many myofascial dysfunctions I was finding. This process was assisted by seeking out alternative manual therapists (e.g., Rolfers) to receive treatment and training. In addition, I was taking many courses on joint mobilization that assisted me to eventually develop the functional mobilization system. However, there are many unique components to the FMT system that have been developed by my wife, Vicky Saliba Johnson, and myself as a direct response to patient problems, knowledge, and intuition. The unique components include the organizational scaffolding that underpins the system, the integrated approach that focuses on enhancing function, and the use of active movement and resistance to perform mobilizations. So to make a long answer short, the impetus was my passion for serving patients, problem-solving, and enhancing function.

What drives your continued growth of this style of therapy, and how is it disparate from traditional physical therapy?

It is difficult to compare our approach to traditional physical therapy because it is difficult to define traditional PT. However, what now drives my continued desire to improve and grow is a passion to offer those I mentor the best options possible for managing their patients. I know, for me, that the ability to successfully manage complex problems in my professional career has enhanced the quality of my personal life. I strongly desire to assist other PTs to have the best tools available serve their patients and to offer each community the option to be treated with the integrated FMT system. In every community where and CFMT therapists or FMT fellows practice, they are recognized for their capacity to treat complex patient problems. The difference is that FMT offers a broad spectrum of tools to manage the mechanical capacity, neuromuscular function, and motor control problems in each patient. These tools include:

- Functional tests that guide the therapist in developing their treatment strategies;
- Manually guided training to facilitate automatic core engagement and efficient movement patterns;
- Integrated self-exercise programs that patients desire to perform;
- Understanding of the interrelated function of the body as a whole;
- A systematic organization of treatment progression;
- Use of patient involved motions and therapist resistance to mobilize restricted structures;
- Application of PNF principles to train new ranges of motions and more efficient movement patterns;

- Training patients to be independent of their therapists; [and]
- Offering ongoing evaluations and treatment to assure the most efficient physical state possible.

Why do you define color and give it a tangible nature in the treatment of your patients?

Utilizing all the patient's senses for their rehabilitation expands our options for effective care. Pain is an experience, which links symptoms to emotions and personal history and decisions. Pain within the medical model is often described as a one-dimensional sensation; however, many individuals, when guided by their therapists, can define their symptoms according to shape (depth and contours), color, and volume of intensity. This process creates a tangible structure for both the therapist and patient to understand and manage the presenting symptoms.

Are you ever surprised by how people assign dimensions to their maladies?

Patients' actions and responses do not surprise me much anymore, but I continue to be intrigued. As much as it is important to be able to scientifically categorize your patient's response, it is also important to recognize that each individual is unique in their response to, their view of, their self-imposed limitations from, and their attitude towards their symptoms. As a therapist, we should thrive on the challenge of understanding each patient's symptoms, history, and response. By striving to enter into each patient's experience, we learn more about our process of management so that we can develop appropriate tools and remain passionate about the care we provide. One of the major challenges of categorizing patients and letting the category direct our care is that the process lent itself to therapist malaise and missed opportunities to learn.

Do you consider FMT an intuitive medical art?

I would not describe FMT as primarily an intuitive approach. FMT is a logical approach combining scientific evidence, anatomy, kinesiology, pathology, and understanding of human motion to assist the therapist in developing a logical treatment strategy. The approach has well-defined strategies for managing dysfunctions of mechanical capacity, neuromuscular facilitation, and motor control, providing specific treatment protocols for each defined dysfunction. However, we mentor that intuition (the ability to understand something immediately, without the need for conscious reasoning) is a natural part of most professions and life. We encourage our therapists to use logic and intuition in an integrated treatment system. Therefore, I view that intuition (innate knowledge) is a valuable component that an experienced therapist can offer his patients. The value of intuition has been extensively researched and validated, and is a talent that we can all develop. The challenge of imparting and teaching these skills is that there are not precise explanations and guidance that can assist a student to explore these talents. The term *tacit knowledge,* or "We can know more than we can tell," describes this component of our experience that is hard to describe and impart.

What three words describe your experience as a therapist?

Blessed, determined, and serving with a vision.

What qualities in Dr. Lin make him an effective PT?

Justin possesses many qualities that make him an effective PT. Most of all, he is determined to develop his manual therapy and communication skills to their optimal potential. He has a passion for excellence and making others' lives better.

What lead him to these qualities?

His passion for life and for serving his patients.